Introduction

In the past few years, policy makers and researchers have given considerable attention to outcomes report cards in health care – public disclosure of information about the patient-background-adjusted health outcomes of individual hospitals and physicians. The health policy community disagrees on the merits of report cards. Supporters of report cards argue that they enable patients to identify the best physicians and hospitals, while simultaneously giving providers powerful incentives to improve quality. Skeptics argue that report cards may encourage providers to "game" the system by avoiding sick and/or seeking healthy patients in the following way. One medically appropriate factor in a provider's decision how to treat a patient is that patient's health status at the time of the onset of illness. At least for report cards on surgical treatments (such as cardiac bypass surgery, or CABG) or nonemergent conditions, this gives providers the opportunity to decline to treat more difficult or complicated patients for valid medical reasons. Even though outcomes report cards generally adjust reported health outcomes for differences in patients' characteristics (for otherwise providers who treat the most serious cases would necessarily appear to have low quality), developers of report cards can only adjust for characteristics that they can observe. Because of the complexity of patient care, providers are likely to have better information on patients' conditions than even the most clinically detailed database. Providers therefore may be able to improve their outcomes report card by selecting patients on the basis of characteristics that are unobservable to the analysts but predictive of good outcomes. Furthermore, report cards may encourage gaming even if providers do not have superior information on patients' conditions (for example, if providers are risk-averse; see Dranove et al. 2003 for an explanation).

Previous empirical research suggests that the debate over outcomes report cards is of more than academic importance. On one hand, Hannan et al. (1994) report that the CABG report card adopted by New York in 1989 played a significant role in the observed decline in that state's in-hospital CABG mortality rate. On the other hand, Dranove et al. (2003) show that the CABG report cards adopted by New York and Pennsylvania in the early 1990s led to higher levels of resource use and to worse health outcomes, particularly for sicker patients. In particular, they find that patients from New York and Pennsylvania admitted to the hospital with a heart attack (AMI) experienced greater growth in rates of hospital expenditures, greater growth in rates of readmission to the hospital with heart failure and recurrent AMI, and (in some specifications) greater growth in mortality, as compared to demographically-similar patients from other states that did not adopt report cards.

Despite the importance of this debate in health care and related contexts like education, little work has sought to investigate whether report cards could be more constructive if designed in a way that reduced the incentives for and the social costs of provider selection behavior. Some report cards have already altered their design to eliminate the feature that is most likely responsible for the provider selection in the New York and Pennsylvania programs – the requirement to report on all patients receiving an elective operative procedure. California, for example, now publishes AMI outcome reports, which because of the emergent nature of a significant fraction of AMIs, are likely to be more difficult to game than their procedure-based counterparts (California OSHPD 2002). Yet, because a significant fraction of AMIs are nonemergent (Ho et al. 1989),

4

even such an illness-based outcomes report card may suffer from the problems associated with selection.

In this paper, I propose an alternative approach: ranking hospitals on the basis of the travel distances of their Medicare patients. Because Medicare is accepted at essentially all US hospitals with equal beneficiary deductibles and copayments, differences in quality are the primary reason why beneficiaries would incur the costs of traveling to a farther versus a nearer hospital. Thus, at least in theory, hospitals that draw patients from farther away would be higher quality than hospitals that draw patients from nearby.

To the extent that this is true empirically, a distance report card could dominate conventional outcomes report cards, by measuring quality of care almost as well but suffering less from selection problems. To see this, decompose measured quality into two components: the portion that is correlated with travel distance, and the portion that is orthogonal. Distance report cards rank only on the portion of quality correlated with distance; conventional report cards rank on both. If hospitals can more easily game the portion orthogonal to distances, and the portion correlated with distances is sufficiently large to powerfully distinguish among hospitals on the basis of quality, then gaming of a distance report card is likely to be less prevalent and less destructive than gaming of an outcomes-based report card.

Gaming is likely to be less prevalent because travel imposes tangible costs on patients, and there is no valid medical reason for selection of patients on the basis of distance. So, avoiding nearby (or attracting far-away) patients is likely to be more difficult than avoiding sick (or attracting healthy) patients. Gaming is likely to be less destructive because the social losses from any selection induced by a distance report card would be likely smaller than the social losses from selection induced by an outcomes report card. Since travel distance is, if anything, negatively correlated with health status before treatment (Capps et al. (2001)), publication of a distance-based report card would, if anything, encourage providers to seek out sicker patients. Given that Dranove et al. (2003) report that the greatest losses from the CABG report cards arise out of avoidance of sicker patients, the distortion of providers' incentives that might occur with a distance-based report card is unlikely to be a serious policy problem.

Finally, rankings on the basis of travel distance offer other advantages over outcomes report cards. In contrast to the unidimensional measures of quality generally contained in even very clinically detailed outcomes report cards, information about patients' willingness to incur travel costs both incorporates attributes of quality other than mortality risk and weights those attributes according to patients' revealed preferences.

The purpose of this paper is to estimate the extent of the correlation between distance and quality in order to investigate the feasibility of a hypothetical distance report card. First, I assess the validity of various types of distance report cards by testing whether hospitals with patient populations who travel farther to obtain care have better patient health outcomes, controlling for differences in patients' health status and other characteristics. I find that the fraction of patients at a hospital who have traveled a long distance is significantly negatively correlated with that hospital's patients' expected mortality from AMI and stroke, holding other factors constant. Second, I compare the ability of a hypothetical distance report card to distinguish confidently among hospitals on the basis of expected mortality to the ability of the California AMI report card. The hypothetical distance-based report card I propose is more powerful than the California AMI outcomes report card at distinguishing high-mortality hospitals from the average hospital, but less powerful than the California AMI report card at distinguishing low-mortality hospitals from the average hospital.

The paper proceeds in three parts. In part I, I describe the data and models I use to investigate the two hypotheses above. Part II discusses the results, and part III concludes with some suggestions for policy reform and further research.

I. Data and Models

Data

I use data from three sources. First, I use comprehensive individual-level longitudinal Medicare claims data from the Centers for Medicare and Medicaid Services (CMS) on the health outcomes and medical utilization of virtually all non-rural elderly fee-for-service Medicare beneficiaries with a new occurrence of heart attack (AMI) in 1994 or 1999 or stroke in 1994. I classify strokes into one of three types (in order of declining seriousness): an event in which a blood vessel in the brain bursts, spilling blood into the spaces surrounding the brain cells (hemorrhagic stroke, primary ICD9 diagnosis code of 434 or 436); an event in which the blood supply to the part of the brain is suddenly interrupted by a blood clot (ischemic stroke, primary ICD9 diagnosis code of 435 or 362.34); and a transient ischemic attack (an ischemic stroke that lasts only a few minutes) or other adverse cerebrovascular event (primary ICD9 diagnosis code of 437). I measure outcomes with five variables: mortality within one year of initial admission (including deaths out of hospital), readmission for subsequent AMI or heart failure (HF) within one year (AMI patients only), and readmission for subsequent stroke or stroke complications (including paralysis, pneumonia, and urinary tract infections) within one year (stroke patients only). Measures of the occurrence of complications were obtained by abstracting data on the principal diagnosis for all subsequent admissions (not counting transfers and readmissions within 30 days of the index admission) in the year following the patient's initial admission. Treatment of AMI patients is intended to prevent subsequent AMIs if possible, and the occurrence of HF requiring hospitalization is evidence that the damage to the patient's heart from ischemic disease has serious functional consequences. I also measure a patient's total hospital utilization with the sum of acute and non-acute (mostly skilled nursing) Medicare expenditures (including deductibles and copayments) in the year following admission for the study illness. Expenditures include all inpatient reimbursements (including copayments and deductibles not paid by Medicare) from insurance claims for all hospitalizations in the year following each patient's initial admission. Data on patient demographic characteristics were obtained from CMS's HISKEW enrollment files, with death dates based on death reports validated by the Social Security Administration.

Second, I use data on U.S. hospital characteristics collected by the American Hospital Association (AHA). The response rate of hospitals to the AHA survey is greater than 90 percent, with response rates above 95 percent for large hospitals (>300 beds). Third, I use a hospital system database constructed from multiple sources (see Madison 2001 for a detailed discussion). The AHA survey contains extensive year-by-year information on hospital system membership status. Validity checking indicated that the universe of systems and system hospitals, and the timing of hospitals' system membership, as defined by AHA did not conform to discussion of hospital systems in the trade press such as Modern Healthcare. We therefore created our own system database based on a combination of the AHA and other sources.

Models

I model the determinants of the intensity of treatment and health outcomes of individual elderly Medicare patients with AMI and stroke. In zip code z lying in MSA of size M_z (M_z is a vector of 5 indicator variables capturing six size categories) during year t = 1994 or 1999, observational units in the analysis consist of individuals i=1,. . ., N_{zt} who are initially admitted to hospital j = 1, ..., J with a new occurrence of illness. Each patient has observable demographic characteristics X_{izt}: four age indicator variables (70-74 years, 75-79 years, 80-89 years, and 90-99 years; omitted group is 65-69 years), gender, and black/nonblack race; and a full set of interaction effects between age, gender, and race. Each patient has health status upon admission to the hospital A_{izt}, where $A_{izt} = 1$ if the patient had acute care hospital utilization in the year prior to his/her illness. The patient then receives treatment that results in Medicare expenditures of R_{izt}. The patient has a health outcome O_{izt}, possibly affected by the intensity of treatment received, where a higher value denotes a more adverse outcome (O is binary in all of our outcome models).

I match to each patient by hospital of admission and year several hospital characteristics (K_{jt}) that may affect treatment and quality of care and are likely to be correlated with the willingness of patients to incur travel costs to attend the hospital: hospital bed size (indicators included for medium (100-300 beds) and large (300+ beds) hospitals, omitted group is small hospitals); hospital teaching status; hospital ownership

9

status (indicators included for for-profit and public ownership, omitted group is nonprofit ownership); whether the hospital had a catheterization (cardiac imaging) laboratory; and whether the hospital was high-volume (more than 75 AMI admissions). In addition, I match by hospital of admission one of five measures of the relative travel distances of that hospital's Medicare patients (L_{jt}), where relative travel distance is defined as the distance from the patient to the hospital divided by the distance from the patient to his or her nearest hospital.[1] These five measures include the 25th percentile of patients' relative travel distances at the hospital; the median patient's relative travel distance at the hospital; the 75th percentile of patients' relative travel distances at the hospital; the fraction of patients at the hospital with a relative travel distance greater than 1 (i.e., for whom the hospital was not the closest choice); and the fraction of patients at the hospital with a relative travel distance greater than 1.5 (i.e., for whom the hospital was at least 150% of the distance to the closest).

I estimate linear models of expenditures and outcomes as a function of 3-digit zip-code-fixed-effects (α_z); year-fixed-effects (θ_t) that vary by MSA size M_z, to capture differences in cost and quality due, for example, to differences in the diffusion of technology in more versus less populous areas; patient demographic characteristics (X_{izt}); health status (A_{izt}); hospital characteristics (K_{jt}); and hospital quality as proxied by relative travel distance (L_{jt}):

$\ln(R_{izt})$

$$O_{izt} \quad = \alpha_z + M_z * \theta_t + X_{izt}\phi + \eta A_{izt} + K_{jt}\gamma + \delta L_{jt} + \epsilon_{izt}, \qquad (1)$$

where ϵ_{izt} is an independently-distributed error term, with $E(\epsilon_{izt} \mid ...) = 0$.

---

[1] To reduce measurement error, patients who chose a hospital within 1 mile of their residence are categorized as having attended their closest hospital, even if there was an alternative hospital which had a calculated distance of less than 1 mile.

II.   Results

Tables 1 and 2 show that a ranking of hospitals based on Medicare beneficiaries' travel distances is negatively correlated with hospitals' average rates of adverse health outcomes and positively correlated with hospitals' average Medicare expenditures. Table 1 presents the average rate of all-cause mortality, cardiac complications, and intensity of treatment for patients with AMI in 1994 and 1999 (N = 285,367) initially admitted to "high-distance" hospitals – those with their median patient's relative travel distance greater than 1 -- and "low-distance" hospitals—those with their median patient's relative travel distance equal to 1. Table 1 analyzes the care of beneficiaries admitted to the hospital separately for patients with and without an inpatient hospital admission in the year before their AMI.

The first column of Table 1 shows that patients who were admitted for AMI to a high-distance hospital experienced better health outcomes than did patients who were admitted to a low-distance hospital. Patients admitted to a high distance hospital experienced .71 percentage points (=33.54 - 34.25), or 2.1 percent (=.71/33.54) lower one-year all-cause mortality than patients admitted to a low-distance hospital. The effect of admission to a high-distance hospital on readmission rates are more mixed, with rates of readmission with AMI slightly lower and rates of readmission with CHF slightly higher, indicating that the additional survivors were not in markedly poor cardiac health. In any event, this result should be interpreted with some caution. Readmission rates measure health outcomes only imperfectly; some readmissions to the hospital may represent a decision to provide additional treatment conditional on health rather than a decline in health.

The second and third columns of Table 1 show that the mortality gain to attending a high-distance hospital was slightly greater for sicker patients, consistent with a model in which the benefits of quality are larger for the more severely ill. PRIOR-ADM measures the health status of a patient prior to admission, where PRIOR-ADM =1 for every patient who had an inpatient hospital admission in the year prior to their admission for AMI (the population mean of PRIOR-ADM is .30). Among those patients who were in good health at the time of their AMI (N= 199,152), those who were admitted to a high-distance hospital experienced .7 percentage points lower mortality. Among those patients who were in poor health at the time of their AMI (N=86,215), those who were admitted to a high-distance hospital experienced .85 percentage points lower mortality. Table 1 also suggests one reason why high-distance hospitals have better outcomes: more intensive treatment. Patients' hospital expenditures in the year after their AMI were 4.9 percent (= (21130-20149) / 20149) higher at high-distance hospitals.

Table 2 presents analogous descriptive statistics on the complications, mortality, health status, and utilization of patients with stroke in 1994 (all strokes, N = 252,742; hemorrhagic strokes, N = 29,460; ischemic strokes, N = 156,260; transient ischemic attack and other cerebrovascular event, N = 67,022). As with AMI patients, mortality of high-distance patients is lower; utilization of high-distance patients is higher; and the health status of high-distance patients is worse. The average mortality gain from admission to a high-distance versus a low-distance hospital is smaller for stroke (.09 percentage points) than for AMI, but the mortality gain from admission to a high-distance hospital for the most severely ill (hemorrhagic) stroke patients, 1.72 percentage points, is substantially larger. However, the larger mortality gain for this population is accompanied by a higher differential rate of readmission with complications. Hemorrhagic stroke patients admitted to a high-distance hospital were .89 percentage points more likely to be readmitted with stroke and .6 percentage points more likely to be readmitted with other complications, as compared to patients admitted to a low-distance hospital. For the reasons above, this result should be interpreted with some caution; readmissions for patients with stroke frequently represent readmission to nonacute facilities for rehabilitation, rather than readmission for treatment of complications.

Consistent with previous work, there is no evidence that patients admitted to high-distance hospitals are healthier than their low-distance-hospital counterparts; if anything, they are slightly sicker. Statistics not presented in Table 1 show that 30.3 percent of patients admitted to a high-distance hospital had an inpatient admission in the year prior to AMI, as compared to 30.1 percent of patients admitted to a low-distance hospital. Patients' prior year expenditures conditional on PRIOR-ADM = 1 were 5.3 percent (= (12668-12031) / 12031) higher for those initially admitted to a high-distance hospital, suggesting that these patients were slightly sicker on admission. Differences in the health status of patients with stroke admitted to high-distance versus low-distance hospitals are similar. Statistics not presented in Table 2 show that 34 percent of patients admitted to a high-distance hospital had an inpatient admission in the year prior to stroke, as compared to 33.9 percent of patients admitted to a low-distance hospital. For this reason, the negative correlation between distance and subsequent health outcomes is not likely due to differences in patients' health status at high-distance versus low-distance hospitals.

Table 3 describes the distributions of the five distance-based measures of hospital quality that I analyze in the regression models that follow. The top panel of the table presents the (patient-weighted) distribution of hospitals' travel distances for AMI patients

from 1994 and 1999; the bottom panel of the table presents the distribution of hospitals'

travel distances for stroke patients. The top three rows of each panel describe the

distribution across hospitals of the distribution of patients' relative travel distances. The

average median relative travel distance is 1.8 – that is, at the average hospital, half the

patients traveled more than 180% of the distance to their closest hospital, and half

traveled less. The average median relative travel distance is larger than the median

median relative travel distance because of a set of hospitals that have very high median

patient travel distances, i.e., attract most of their patients from afar. According to the

bottom two rows of each panel, the fraction of patients at a hospital for whom the

hospital was not their closest is distributed uniformly. For AMI patients, the mean

(median) of the distribution is .5, the 10th percentile is .1, and the 90th percentile is .91.

For stroke patients, the distribution is slightly heavier at the top of the distribution (higher

mean and bottom quantiles, lower top quantiles). Not surprisingly, using a more stringent

definition of high-distance hospital (i.e., classifying a hospital as high-distance if it was at

least 150% of the distance to the patient's closest hospital) shifts the distribution

downward roughly proportionately.

Tables 4 and 5 present estimates of δ from equation (1) for patients with AMI and

stroke, respectively. The top three rows of table 4 present estimates of the effect of the

25th percentile, median, and 75th percentile of a hospital's AMI patients' travel distance

on mortality, cardiac complications, and Medicare expenditures. The estimated effects of

these three quantiles of a hospital's patients' relative travel distance on both outcomes

and expenditures are small and statistically insignificant. The bottom two rows of Table

4 present estimates of the effect of the proportion of AMI patients at a hospital for whom the hospital was high-distance, where a high-distance hospital is defined either as a hospital that is not a patient's closest hospital or as a hospital that is at least 150% of the distance to a patient's closest hospital. These two measures of patient travel distance are significantly negatively correlated with adverse outcomes and positively correlated with expenditures. Moving from a hospital that was the closest choice for all of its patients to a hospital that was the closest choice for none of its patients leads, in expectation, to 1.03 percentage points lower mortality and approximately 2.9 percent higher Medicare expenditures, holding other factors constant. These effects are of the same order of magnitude as the raw differences in Table 1. Using the more stringent definition of a high-distance hospital leads to greater mortality and expenditure effects. The effects of these measures of travel distance on complications rates are small and statistically insignificant.

Moving an AMI patient from a low-distance to a high-distance hospital is a cost-effective way to improve quality of care. For example, moving a patient from a hospital that was the closest choice for all versus none of its patients leads to an increase in Medicare expenditures of approximately \$632 (=.0286*\$22,119 average 1999 AMI Medicare expenditures) and a decrease in mortality of 1.03 percentage points, which implies that the additional treatment at high-distance versus low-distance hospitals is efficient assuming a cost per year of life saved of at least \$61,419 (=632/.0103). This is well below the value of an added year of life that would be inferred from most published studies (Viscusi 1993; Duke University Center for Health Policy, Law, and Management 2004). Using the more stringent definition of a high-distance hospital leads to virtually the same implied cost-effectiveness of treatment at a high-distance versus low-distance hospital. The same implied cost-effectiveness ratios hold for the additional treatment obtained by moving a patient to an incrementally higher-distance hospital, although the absolute expenditure increase and mortality decrease is smaller (multiply numerator and denominator of ratio by an arbitrarily small number ω).

Table 5 presents estimates of the effect of the proportion of stroke patients at each hospital for whom the hospital was high distance on the outcomes and expenditures for stroke. The top panel of table 5 presents estimates of the effect of travel distance on all stroke patients grouped together; the bottom three panels present estimates for each type of stroke patient separately. The effects of travel distance on stroke patients' outcomes and Medicare expenditures are larger than the effect of distance on AMI patients. According to the top panel of the table, moving from a hospital that was high distance for none versus all of its patients leads, in expectation, to 1.1 to 1.83 percentage points lower stroke mortality, and to approximately 5.1 to 7.4 percent higher Medicare expenditures, holding other factors constant. In cost-effectiveness terms, moving a stroke patient from a hospital at which none versus all of its patients were high-distance leads to additional Medicare treatments that are efficient assuming a value per year of life saved of at least $68,212 (=.0737*$16,937/.0183), which is very similar to the effect for AMI. For patients with transient ischemic attack and other adverse cerebrovascular events, choice of hospital based on its patients' travel distance translates into a maximum mortality gain of 13 percent (= 1.75 / 13.45 percentage points average mortality) which is substantial. This mortality effect is especially striking given that it is accompanied by a decreased rate of subsequent readmission for stroke and by insignificantly higher Medicare

16

expenditures. In other words, moving a patient with transient ischemic attack to a higher-distance hospital is necessarily welfare-improving. For sicker (hemorrhagic) stroke patients, the substantial mortality gain of admission to a high-distance hospital is accompanied by an increased rate of readmission rate both for stroke and for other complications, indicating that they may be in more marginal health. However, in results not presented in the table, if the readmission variables are defined to exclude all nonacute care hospital (largely skilled nursing) admissions, the estimated effect of distance on readmission declines and becomes statistically insignificant. Because nonacute admission after stroke may measure both the existence of complications and the supply of additional services conditional on health status, this finding mitigates the negative implications of the estimated effect of distance on complications in this population.

In order to investigate whether the estimated effects of a hospital's patients' travel distance are due to unobserved differences in patients' health status, I estimated δ with instrumental variables (IV) methods, using as instruments functions of patients' distances to high-distance hospitals. Intuitively, these methods compare the outcomes of patients who live nearby to a high-distance hospital versus those who live far away from one. Under the assumption that patient residential location decisions are uncorrelated with their health status, IV estimates of the effect of treatment at a high-distance hospital will be consistent, regardless of differences in the characteristics of patients who are actually treated at high-distance versus low-distance hospitals.

I experimented with several different specifications. One specification used as instruments the proportion of patients at the nearest hospital for whom the hospital was not the closest choice; the relative distance to the nearest hospital that was not the closest choice (i.e., the distance to the nearest high-distance hospital divided by the distance to the nearest hospital) for at least 75 percent its patients; the relative distance to the nearest hospital that was not the closest choice for at least 50 percent of its patients; and the relative distance to the nearest hospital that was not the closest choice for at least 25 percent of its patients. An alternative specification estimated the effect of admission to a hospital that was not the closest choice for at least 50 percent of its patients, using as an instrument each patient's relative distance to the nearest hospital that was not the closest choice for at least 50 percent of its patients. Estimates of δ from these models were very sensitive to choice of specification and had generally large standard errors

Table 6 investigates the second key concern about distance-based report cards: can they distinguish confidently between hospitals on the basis of quality? For each of the five patient populations I examine (AMI, all stroke, and three types of strokes separately), table 6 reports the expected deviation from average mortality for a patient admitted to hospitals of different qualities, and the 98 percent confidence intervals around the expected deviations. The first column of the table reproduces the estimate of δ from equation (1) from tables 4 and 5. The second column reports the expected mortality for a reference patient admitted to the hospital at the 10th percentile of the distribution, i.e., the 10th percentile of the quality measure*δ, less the expected mortality for a reference patient admitted to the average hospital, with upper and lower 98 percent confidence intervals. The third column reports the expected mortality for a reference patient admitted to the hospital at the 90th percentile of the distribution less the expected mortality for a reference patient admitted to the average hospital.

Table 6 shows that a hypothetical distance report card can distinguish confidently the worst decile of hospitals from the average hospital. For every patient population and each of the two distance measures, the lower bound of the 98 percent confidence interval around the expected deviation from average mortality for a patient admitted to the 10th percentile hospital is greater than zero. In fact, for AMI patients, calculations not in table 6 show that the lower bound of the 98 percent confidence interval around the expected deviation from average mortality for a patient admitted to the 25th percentile hospital is greater than zero as well. The hypothetical distance report card is less able to powerfully distinguish the best hospitals from the average hospital. For no patient population is the upper bound of the 98 percent confidence interval around the expected deviation from average mortality for a patient admitted to the 90th percentile hospital less than zero.

In comparison to the California AMI outcomes report card, the hypothetical distance-based report card I propose is more powerful at distinguishing low-quality hospitals from the average hospital, but less powerful at distinguishing high-quality hospitals from the average hospital. According to the table on page 16 of the 1996-98 report (California OSHPD 2002), the AMI outcomes report card found that 8.0 percent of hospitals had risk-adjusted mortality rates that were better than expected in at least one model, and 10.6 percent of hospitals had risk-adjusted mortality rates that were worse than expected in at least one model. This is the same as the number of hospitals in the report for which the upper (lower) bound of the 98 percent confidence interval of the risk-adjusted mortality rate fell below (above) the state average. In other words, the California AMI outcomes report card can distinguish the top 8.0 percent and the bottom 10.6 percent of hospitals from the mean. The hypothetical distance-based report card can distinguish confidently up to the 25th percentile from the mean; however, it can not

confidently distinguish the top decile (or even the top 8 percent of hospitals) from the

mean.

III. Conclusion

How useful would be a hospital report card based on patients' travel distances? A

report card based on patients' willingness to travel for treatment could dominate

conventional outcomes report cards, if it suffered less from selection problems but

measured quality at least as well. Although the theoretical case for a distance report card

on grounds of selection is clear, the ability of a distance report card to measure quality is

an unresolved empirical issue. For a distance report card to be useful in practice, it would

need to be both valid – that is, correlated with true quality – and able to distinguish

confidently among hospitals – that is, able to reject at conventional significance levels the

hypothesis that the true quality of a low-ranked hospital was the same as the quality of

the average hospital.

In this paper, I propose a specific distance report card, and document empirically

that it would be both valid and powerful. I assign to each non-rural general

medical/surgical hospital in the US a ranking based on the fraction of Medicare patients

at the hospital with one or more specific illnesses for whom the hospital was not their

closest choice (and variants of this, such as the fraction of patients for whom the hospital

was at least 150% of the distance to their closest choice). I use longitudinal claims data

on elderly Medicare beneficiaries admitted to the hospital with cardiac and

cerebrovascular illnesses in 1994 and 1999, matched with data on the characteristics of all general medical/surgical hospitals. These data include information on each patients'

demographic characteristics, type and severity of illness on admission to the hospital,

subsequent Medicare expenditures, and health outcomes, measured by all-cause one-year

mortality and readmission to the hospital with complications.

I report four key findings. First, hospitals with patient populations who travel

farther to obtain care have statistically significantly better outcomes, holding other factors

constant. For example, for a patient with heart attack, moving from a hospital that was

the closest choice for all of its patients to a hospital that was the closest choice for none

of its patients leads, in expectation, to about a percentage point significantly lower

mortality with no measurable increase in cardiac complications – a small, but nontrivial

effect.

Second, the implied cost-effectiveness of the incremental treatment at a high-

distance versus a low-distance hospital is high by conventional standards. The better

outcomes at high-distance versus low-distance hospitals are due in part to more intensive

treatment; at least for some populations, patients admitted to high-distance hospitals have

slightly higher average Medicare expenditures in the year following their illness than do

patients admitted to low-distance hospitals. For AMI and stroke patients in aggregate,

moving from a hospital at which none to one at which all of its patients were high-

distance leads to additional Medicare treatments that are efficient assuming a value per

year of life saved of $60,000 to $70,000 – by conventional standards, a low threshold to

meet. Furthermore, for less severely ill patients with stroke (those with transient

ischemic attack and other adverse cerebrovascular events), choice of hospital based on its

patients' travel distance translates into a mortality gain of 13 percent (= 1.75 percentage points/ 13.45) percentage points average mortality) which is substantial. This mortality effect is especially striking given that it is accompanied by a decreased rate of subsequent readmission for stroke and by insignificantly higher Medicare expenditures. At least for these patients, choice of hospital based on distance would be unambiguously welfare-improving.

Third, there is no evidence that the better outcomes of patients at high-distance hospitals are due to more their favorable health status on admission; if anything, the opposite is (weakly) true. Patients admitted to a high distance hospital are slightly more likely to have had an inpatient admission in the year prior to the onset of illness, and conditional on an admission, had higher Medicare hospital expenditure during that prior year.

Fourth, a hypothetical distance report card can distinguish confidently the worst hospitals from the average hospital. For every patient population and each of the two distance measures, the lower bound of the 98 percent confidence interval around the expected deviation from average mortality for a patient admitted to the 10th percentile hospital is greater than zero. For AMI patients, moreover, a distance-based report card can distinguish the bottom quarter of hospitals from the average. The hypothetical distance report card is less able to powerfully distinguish the best hospitals from the average hospital, although from a policy perspective, this may be less important. This compares favorably to (although does not necessarily dominate) existing outcomes report cards, such as the California AMI outcomes report card. According to the California Office of Statewide Health Planning and Development, the AMI outcomes report card can confidently distinguish the top 8.0 percent and the bottom 10.6 percent of hospitals from the mean.

For these reasons, I conclude that distance based report cards can serve as a useful measure of hospital quality. Future research might explore the power of other distance-based reporting mechanisms and the validity and power of using distance report cards for other illnesses and other patient populations.

Table 1: Health outcomes, health expenditures, and health on admission of elderly medicare beneficiaries with AMI
Admitted to high-distance and low-distance hospitals, 1994 and 1999
All patients and those with and without an inpatient admission in the year prior to AMI

	Total	Good health on admission: PRIOR-ADM = 0	Poor health on admission: PRIOR-ADM = 1
365 day mortality			
High Distance Hospital	33.54%	29.23%	43.44%
Low Distance Hospital	34.25%	29.93%	44.29%
365 day CHF readmission			
High Distance Hospital	8.75%	6.95%	12.86%
Low Distance Hospital	8.61%	6.85%	12.68%
365 day AMI readmission			
High Distance Hospital	5.44%	4.75%	7.03%
Low Distance Hospital	5.56%	4.95%	6.96%
365 day prior to admission inpatient expenditures			
High Distance Hospital	$3,844	$0	$12,668
Low Distance Hospital	$3,618	$0	$12,031
365 day total inpatient expenditures			
High Distance Hospital	$21,130	$20,562	$22,433
Low Distance Hospital	$20,149	$19,805	$20,949

Table 2: Health outcomes, health expenditures, and health on admission of elderly Medicare beneficiaries with stroke Admitted to high-distance and low-distance hospitals, 1994

	All strokes	Hemorrhagic Strokes	Occlusive Strokes	Transient Ischemic Attack/Other
365 day mortality				
High Distance Hospital	29.67%	51.85%	32.19%	13.19%
Low Distance Hospital	29.76%	53.57%	32.58%	13.76%
365 day Stroke readmission				
High Distance Hospital	15.00%	13.46%	16.10%	13.13%
Low Distance Hospital	14.79%	12.57%	15.70%	13.59%
365 day Other Complication Readmission				
High Distance Hospital	7.36%	6.61%	8.03%	6.13%
Low Distance Hospital	7.25%	5.96%	7.86%	6.38%
365 day prior to admission inpatient expenditures				
High Distance Hospital	$4,059	$3,734	$3,899	$4,593
Low Distance Hospital	$3,802	$3,511	$3,656	$4,255
365 day total inpatient expenditures				
High Distance Hospital	$17,411	$21,892	$19,032	$11,462
Low Distance Hospital	$16,327	$20,026	$17,977	$11,052

**Table 3: Patient-weighted distributions
of hospitals' distance-based quality measures for
elderly Medicare beneficiaries with AMI and stroke, 1994-1999**

	Average	10th percentile	Median	90th percentile
AMI, 1994 and 1999				
25th pctile of relative travel distance of patients at your hospital	1.18	1.00	1.00	1.60
Median relative travel distance of patients at your hospital	1.82	1.00	1.02	2.57
75th pctile of relative travel distance of patients at your hospital	4.14	1.00	1.91	6.57
Fraction of patients at your hospital for whom hospital was not their closest	50.6%	10.2%	50.0%	91.4%
Fraction of patients at your hospital for whom hospital was > 150% of distance to their closest	38.7%	7.1%	34.6%	78.1%
Stroke, 1994				
25th pctile of relative travel distance of patients at your hospital	1.18	1.00	1.00	1.50
Median relative travel distance of patients at your hospital	1.79	1.00	1.11	2.64
75th pctile of relative travel distance of patients at your hospital	4.21	1.00	2.21	6.88
Fraction of patients at your hospital for whom hospital was not their closest	52.9%	13.5%	53.9%	90.3%
Fraction of patients at your hospital for whom hospital was > 150% of distance to their closest	38.5%	9.2%	36.5%	71.2%

Table 4: Effect of distance-based hospital quality measures on health outcomes and health expenditures of elderly Medicare beneficiaries with AMI, 1994 and 1999 (standard errors in parentheses)

	1year mortality	1year AMI readmit rate	1year CHF readmit rate	Ln(1yr total expenditure)
25th pctile of relative travel distance of patients at your hospital	0.05 (0.05)	-0.01 (0.02)	0.00 (0.03)	0.16 (0.10)
Median relative travel distance of patients at your hospital	0.00 (0.01)	0.00 (0.01)	0.00 (0.01)	0.01 (0.03)
75th pctile of relative travel distance of patients at your hospital	0.01 (0.01)	0.00 (0.00)	0.00 (0.00)	0.02 (0.01)
Fraction of patients at your hospital for whom hospital was not their closest	-1.03 (0.38)	-0.31 (0.19)	0.00 (0.23)	2.86 (0.85)
Fraction of patients at your hospital for whom hospital was > 150% of distance to their closest	-1.33 (0.41)	-0.25 (0.21)	0.13 (0.25)	3.67 (0.92)

Table 5: Effect of distance-based hospital quality measures on health outcomes and health expenditures of elderly Medicare beneficiaries with stroke, 1994 (standard errors in parentheses)

	1year mortality	1year stroke readmit rate	1year other complication readmit rate	Ln(1yr total expenditure)
All Strokes				
Fraction of patients at your hospital for whom hospital was not their closest	-1.10 (0.41)	-0.08 (0.34)	0.14 (0.25)	5.05 (0.88)
Fraction of patients at your hospital for whom hospital was > 150% of distance to their closest	-1.83 (0.50)	0.11 (0.41)	0.25 (0.30)	7.37 (1.06)
Hemorrhagic Strokes				
Fraction of patients at your hospital for whom hospital was not their closest	-2.93 (1.44)	1.57 (0.99)	0.96 (0.71)	12.31 (2.79)
Fraction of patients at your hospital for whom hospital was > 150% of distance to their closest	-4.17 (1.70)	2.48 (1.16)	1.59 (0.84)	19.65 (3.29)
Occlusive Strokes				
Fraction of patients at your hospital for whom hospital was not their closest	-0.87 (0.56)	0.28 (0.45)	0.11 (0.33)	5.56 (1.08)
Fraction of patients at your hospital for whom hospital was > 150% of distance to their closest	-1.49 (0.67)	0.36 (0.54)	0.14 (0.40)	6.86 (1.30)
Transient Ischemic Attack/Other				
Fraction of patients at your hospital for whom hospital was not their closest	-0.93 (0.62)	-1.51 (0.63)	-0.03 (0.45)	1.04 (1.77)
Fraction of patients at your hospital for whom hospital was > 150% of distance to their closest	-1.75 (0.75)	-1.53 (0.76)	-0.07 (0.54)	2.55 (2.14)

Table 6: Expected deviation from average mortality for a patient admitted to hospitals of various qualities, elderly Medicare beneficiaries with AMI and stroke
(standard errors in parentheses)
[98 percent confidence intervals in brackets]

	Estimated effect of a unit change in quality index (standard error) from table 4-5	Expected deviation from average mortality for a patient admitted to…	
		The 10th percentile hospital [confidence interval]	The 90th percentile hospital [confidence interval]
AMI			
Fraction of patients at your hospital for whom hospital was not their closest	-1.03 (0.38)	0.41 [0.32,0.50]	-0.42 [-1.23,0.38]
Fraction of patients at your hospital for whom hospital was > 150% of distance to their closest	-1.33 (0.41)	0.42 [0.35,0.48]	-0.53 [-1.27,0.21]
All Strokes			
Fraction of patients at your hospital for whom hospital was not their closest	-1.10 (0.41)	0.43 [0.30,0.56]	-0.41 [-1.27,0.45]
Fraction of patients at your hospital for whom hospital was > 150% of distance to their closest	-1.83 (0.50)	0.53 [0.42,0.64]	-0.60 [-1.43,0.22]
Hemorrhagic Strokes			
Fraction of patients at your hospital for whom hospital was not their closest	-2.93 (1.44)	1.16 [0.64,1.67]	-1.07 [-4.12,1.99]
Fraction of patients at your hospital for whom hospital was > 150% of distance to their closest	-4.17 (1.70)	1.27 [0.86,1.68]	-1.42 [-4.37,1.53]
Occlusive Strokes			
Fraction of patients at your hospital for whom hospital was not their closest	-0.87 (0.56)	0.35 [0.18,0.52]	-0.33 [-1.50,0.85]
Fraction of patients at your hospital for whom hospital was > 150% of distance to their closest	-1.49 (0.67)	0.43 [0.29,0.58]	-0.49 [-1.59,0.62]
Transient Ischemic Attack/Other			
Fraction of patients at your hospital for whom hospital was not their closest	-0.93 (0.62)	0.36 [0.17,0.56]	-0.35 [-1.64,0.95]
Fraction of patients at your hospital for whom hospital was > 150% of distance to their closest	-1.75 (0.75)	0.51 [0.35,0.67]	-0.56 [-1.78,0.66]

References

California Office of Statewide Health Planning and Development (OSHPD), California Hospital Outcomes Project, "Heart Attack Outcomes: 1996-98," (2002) http://www.oshpd.state.ca.us/HQAD/HIRC/hospital/Outcomes/HeartAttacks/, accessed April 10, 2004.

Dranove, David, Daniel Kessler, Mark McClellan, and Mark Satterthwaite, "Is More Information Better? The Effects of 'Report Cards' on Health Care Providers," *Journal of Political Economy* 111 (2003), pp. 555-88.

Capps, Cory S., David Dranove, Share Greenstein, and Mark Satterthwaite, "The Silent Majority Fallacy of the Elzing-Hogarty Criteria: A Critique and New Approach to Analyzing Hospital Mergers," NBER Working Paper 8216 (2001).

Duke University Center for Health Policy, Law, and Management, "Willingness to Pay per Added Year of Life, United States, 1993," www.hpolicy.duke.edu/cyberexchange/wtpvalue1.pdf, accessed April 10, 2004.

Hannan, Edward L. et al., "Improving the Outcomes of Coronary Artery Bypass Surgery in New York State," *Journal of the American Medical Association* 271 (March 9, 1994), pp. 761-66.

Ho, Mary T. et al, "Delay Between Onset of Chest Pain and Seeking Medicare Care: The Effect of Public Education," *Annals of Emergency Medicine* 187 (July 1989), pp. 727-31.

Madison, Kristin, "The Relationship Between Multihospital System Membership and Treatments, Costs, and Outcomes of Medicare Patients with Acute Myocardial Infarction," PhD. Thesis, Stanford University (2001).

Viscusi, W. Kip, "The Value of Risks to Life and Health," *Journal of Economic Literature* 31 (December 1993), pp. 1912-46.